Kakooza Abdul Wahabu
Lamwaka Melat Linda
Nakato Agnes Anitah

Neonatal Hygiene among Breastfeeding Mother

AF757274

Kakooza Abdul Wahabu
Lamwaka Melat Linda
Nakato Agnes Anitah

Neonatal Hygiene among Breastfeeding Mother

Knowledge and Practices on Neonatal Hygiene among Breastfeeding Mothers

LAP LAMBERT Academic Publishing

Imprint

Any brand names and product names mentioned in this book are subject to trademark, brand or patent protection and are trademarks or registered trademarks of their respective holders. The use of brand names, product names, common names, trade names, product descriptions etc. even without a particular marking in this work is in no way to be construed to mean that such names may be regarded as unrestricted in respect of trademark and brand protection legislation and could thus be used by anyone.

Cover image: www.ingimage.com

Publisher:
LAP LAMBERT Academic Publishing
is a trademark of
Dodo Books Indian Ocean Ltd. and OmniScriptum S.R.L publishing group

120 High Road, East Finchley, London, N2 9ED, United Kingdom
Str. Armeneasca 28/1, office 1, Chisinau MD-2012, Republic of Moldova, Europe
Managing Directors: Ieva Konstantinova, Victoria Ursu
info@omniscriptum.com

Printed at: see last page
ISBN: 978-620-8-44169-2

Copyright © Kakooza Abdul Wahabu, Lamwaka Melat Linda, Nakato Agnes Anitah
Copyright © 2025 Dodo Books Indian Ocean Ltd. and OmniScriptum S.R.L publishing group

Knowledge and Practices on Neonatal Hygiene among Breastfeeding Mothers at a General Hospital.

Abdul Wahabu Kakooza[1], Agnes Nakato[1], Hope Kyomugisha[1], Melat Linda Lamwaka[1], Edwin Kigozi[2], Elizabeth Namukombe Ekong[1].

Author affiliations

1Uganda Christian University, P.O. Box 4, Mukono, Uganda.

2School of Public Health, Makerere University, P.O. Box 7072, Kampala, Uganda.

Corresponding author:

Abdul Wahabu Kakooza

Uganda Christian University, P.O. Box 4, Mukono, Uganda.

Email: kakoozaabdulwahabu03@gmail.com

Phone number: +256 743069409

Contents

Introduction

Every day, approximately 6,500 newborns lose their lives worldwide, representing 47% of all child deaths under the age of 5. Since 1990, significant progress has been made in improving child survival, with neonatal deaths decreasing from 5 million in 1990 to 2.3 million in 2022(WHO, 2020, 2024). Despite global declines in neonatal mortality over the last decades, rates in most of sub-Saharan Africa have remained largely unchanged. Low- and middle-income countries bear the brunt of this crisis, accounting for 98% of perinatal deaths. Early neonatal deaths represent three-quarters of all neonatal fatalities, with 30% to 50% occurring on the first day of life. A significant portion of these deaths is linked to maternal hygiene (Annettee Nakimuli, 2015).

As of 2022, Uganda's neonatal mortality rate stands at 22 deaths per 1,000 live births(UDHS, 2023), approximating about 45,000 newborns dying each year positioning Uganda as the fifth highest in sub-Saharan Africa for newborn deaths and mortality among children under five, largely attributed to inadequate hygiene practices among breastfeeding mothers(Jacob Sandberg, 2014).

Neonatal Hygiene is a determinant of the newborn care that plays an important role in infant morbidity and mortality worldwide. Proper hygiene practices among lactating mothers are necessary to prevent infection ad ensure the health growth of neonates. Despite the recognized importance of neonatal hygiene, studies indicate varying level of knowledge and practice among mothers, particularly in resource limited settings. A

Karachi based study quantified newborn care behavior and knowledge among mothers attending a tertiary health care Centre. The study revealed gaps in essential neonatal hygiene practices such as cord care and initiation of lactation, which reflect the need for greater maternal education on these issues(Saadia Gul, 2014).

Similarly, in Hossana town of Ethiopia, a survey measured mothers' newborn care practices among one month old infants. Findings were that 30.8% of the months had expected neonatal care practices like early initiation of breastfeeding, cord care, and thermal care. It was found that the assessment that education status and knowledge of mothers played a critical determining role in having proper neonatal hygiene (Amanuel Nuramo Sakelo, 2020).

Based on the hypothesis that increased neonatal mortality is associated with poor hygiene among breast feeding mothers, this study intended to assess the breastfeeding mother's knowledge and practices on neonatal hygiene so as to address a gap in the knowledge and practices on hygiene of breastfeeding mothers towards their neonates. This will provide important information to the breastfeeding mothers, health workers, and other relevant stakeholders that can be used in development of strategies to address concerns surrounding neonatal morbidity and mortality.

Methods

Study Design

This was a mixed study design with both quantitative and qualitative descriptive cross-sectional study.

Study Site

The study was conducted at the post-natal clinic of Mukono General Hospital in Butebe village, Mukono District, Uganda. Mukono general hospital is located in the east of Kampala city along Kampala-Jinja highway approximately 21 kilometers from Kampala the capital city of Uganda. This hospital is owned and operated by the Government of Uganda, through the Uganda's Ministry of Health and offers free services to counties of Goma, Kasawo, Nabaale, Nama, Kkome islands, Kyampisi, Nagojje, Ntenjeru, Kimenyedde, Mukono TC, Nakisunga and Ntunda, and Seeta covering a total population of 932,672(UDHS, 2015).

Study Population

Breastfeeding mothers having children of 28 days of life and below were enrolled into the study.

Selection criteria

Mothers above 18 years of age and breastfeeding babies at 28 days of life and below and willing to participate were included in the study. Those who were absent during data collection, mentally unstable and unwilling to participate were excluded from this study.

Sampling Method

A mixed-method study involving both quantitative and qualitative approaches was used. Simple random sampling with replacement was applied in the quantitative component to ensure that all participants had an equal chance of being selected each time. For the qualitative component, focus group discussions and in-depth interviews were conducted. A convenience sampling method was used, where only mothers present on the day of data collection were considered and then randomized.

Sample Size Determination

Sample size was determined using Kish and Leslie formula cite kish 1965.

$$no = \frac{z^2 pq}{e^2}$$

no – desired sample size

Z – Was the z value at 95% confidence interval, 1.96

p – 95% (0.95)- the estimated number of breastfeeding mothers with the babies below 28 days of life, according Sr. Alex Namara the Senior Nursing Officer of Mukono General Hospital.

q – Is the target population estimated to have characteristics not being measured Q= (1-p) also estimated at 5%and the level of precision level is e - standard error, 0.05

$$no = \frac{1.96^2 \times 0.95 \times 0.05}{0.05^2}$$

no= 73 participants.

Limited time was offered to us by the hospital for data collection due to the COVID-19 Pandemic (One week: November 23rd to 27th, 2020), yet this study was needed in partial fulfillment of academic requirements. Therefore only 30 participants who met the inclusion criteria were recruited for quantitative study.

Data Collection Method

Data for the current study were collected within a period of one week using both qualitative and quantitative methods. For the quantitative component, organized questionnaires were administered to participants who were sampled using simple random sampling with replacement to ensure equal chances of participation. The survey tool was adapted from a quantitative cross-sectional study titled "Assessment of Practices and Knowledge of Breastfeeding Mothers on Maternal and Child Health in Rural Sierra Leone"(Joseph Sam Kanu, 2014) . Permission to use the tool was requested through email, and permission was granted. The standardized questionnaire included closed and open-ended questions, segregated into sections on demographic profile, antenatal history, postnatal and breastfeeding history, knowledge and hygiene practices of lactating mothers, and support obtained from employers, family members, friends, and healthcare providers. The questionnaires were completed by the researchers and in the waiting area of the postnatal clinic, taking approximately 10 to 15 minutes per respondent.

For the qualitative component, data were gathered through in-depth interviews (IDIs) and focus group discussions (FGDs). Convenience sampling was used, targeting only mothers present on the day of data collection. The mothers were then randomly assigned to IDIs or FGDs. All participants provided informed consent before any interview began. The interviews and conversations were conducted both in Luganda and English, the most common languages of the target group, to allow for understanding and comfort. The sessions were conducted in quiet, intimate rooms to maintain confidentiality, and audio-recorded with consent for transcription and thematic analysis.

Reliability and Validity

To ensure high levels of reliability, accuracy, and validity, various quality control measures were employed throughout the study. Pilot testing was conducted prior to actual data collection to test for clarity, acceptability, and relevance of the data collection instruments. The pilot was conducted at Mukono Church of Uganda Hospital, which shared similar community characteristics with the main study site. The pilot allowed the researchers to find out about the hygiene behavior of breastfeeding mothers in handling their neonates. The participants for the pilot study were health-seeking mothers who were breastfeeding, and data from the questionnaires were analyzed using SPSS. Pilot feedback informed modifications that were made to enhance the questionnaire for clarity and contextuality.

Throughout the initial data collection phase, quality of data was also maintained by regular monitoring and review in the field by the principal investigator. All data collected were examined thoroughly for accuracy, consistency, and completeness after each field visit. Questionnaires with more than 10% missing values were not analyzed. Regular debriefing was done on a daily basis with the research team before each data collection session to address any problems and make adjustments as necessary. Data were coded and saved in an Access spreadsheet database for storage and initial analysis. Audio recording of qualitative data was transcribed verbatim, and transcripts were verified for accuracy. All these efforts cumulatively ensured that the data collected were reliable, valid, and representative of the study objectives.

Data Analysis

Data analysis for the mixed methods study was conducted on quantitative and qualitative data to provide a general insight into the purpose of the research. Quantitative data was analyzed using the Statistical Package for the Social Sciences (SPSS) version 24.0. Descriptive analysis was conducted to provide descriptions of the characteristics of all mothers and their babies in the sample. The demographic variables of the mothers including age, educational level, marital status, and employment status were compared using measures of central tendency such as mean and mode, and presented in frequency tables. Antenatal and postnatal history of the pregnancy in question, including health-seeking behavior and whether or not mothers received health education regarding breastfeeding, were summarized by calculating the proportion of mothers who reported being provided with such information by health workers. Knowledge about lactating women's hygiene was scored as a percentage of women who could name at least one maternal or infant benefit of being clean. The knowledge was compared with maternal demographic status, including age and education level. Hygiene habits such as hand washing prior to breastfeeding and breast cleaning were also described and compared with demographic status in an effort to identify trends and patterns. Where it was appropriate, cross-tabulations were used to explore variable relationships, and results were presented using tables and graphs.

Qualitative data were examined using thematic content analysis. Transcripts of verbatim audio-recorded responses were read multiple times to familiarize themselves with the data. Codes were taken from the transcripts and categorized and coded into themes based on patterns emerging. These themes were utilized in interpreting participants' experiences, perceptions, and practices concerning hygiene and breastfeeding. A few quotes were used to authenticate the findings and give voice to the participants. Synthesis of qualitative and quantitative data was carried out at the interpretation stage so that comparison and synthesis of findings could be performed to make more significant and holistic conclusions.

Data Ethical Consideration

An introduction letter to conduct the study was obtained from the nursing department under the faculty of health sciences at Uganda Christian University and was presented to hospital administration of Mukono general hospital.

Each participant signed a consent form to take part in our study. The participants voluntarily participated and confidentiality was maintained throughout the study and the questionnaires were kept in lock and key. For the recording from the interviews and focused group discussions, they kept in one folder and locked on the desktop. The laptop with raw data from the qualitative data collection has a password to ensure protection of the data collected from the patients. After data collection, mothers were given health education concerning the benefits of breastfeeding and hygiene.

Results

This chapter presents the results of the study according to the study objectives.

Results were presented in tables, figures and the explained details are in texts. For most findings, tables have been used in the presentation of the gathered information. A total of 30 respondents for qualitative study, 10mothers were interviewed through qualitative study with 3 group focused discission during the period of data collection yielding 100% response rate.

Socio Demographic Information

Table 1: Socio-demographic information of the study respondents

Demographic data

Variable item	Frequency	Percentage	Mean	Standard deviation
Age			24.9333	4.94754
15-19	5	16.7		
20-24	11	36.7		
25-29	8	26.7		
30-34	5	16.7		
34-39	1	3.3		
Total	30	100		
Buganda	13	43.3		
Ankole	4	13.3		
Busoga	5	16.7		

Iteso	1	3.3
Others	7	23.3
Total	30	100
Primary level	8	26.7
O-level	12	40.0
A-level	6	20.0
Degree level	2	6.7
Not applicable	2	6.7
Total	30	100
Cannot read at all	7	23.3
Able to read part of sentence	6	20.0
Able to read whole sentence	17	56.7

Total	30	100

Table 1 above indicates that majority of the respondents were in age range of 20 to 24years 36.7% (11/30) with a mean age of 24.9333 and standard deviation of 4.9475, 43.3%(13/30) were from the Buganda region while 93.3% (28/30) of them managed to at least attend one or more than one level of education based on Uganda's ministry of education curriculum and 6.7% (2/30) did not manage to attend school at any level. The highest percentage of participants were able to read and understand a whole sentence in English 56.7% (17/30), 20.0% (6/30) were able to read half sentences and the 23.3% (7/30) were unable to read and understand sentences in English.

Pregnancy and Antenatal care

Table 2 indicating the mother's experience in their pregnancy, antenatal and childbirth

Variable items	Frequency	Percentage (%)
Where did the delivery occur? Husband's home	2	6.7
Parent's home	1	3.3
Someone else's home	1	3.3

Traditional birth attendant	1	3.3
Hospital	25	83.3
Total	30	100
Who attended delivery? Midwife	21	70.0
Doctor	3	10.0
Traditional birth attendant	2	6.7
Others	4	13.3
Total	30	100
What was used to cut the baby's cord? Razor blade	20	66.7
Household knife	2	6.7
Scissors	7	23.3
Others	1	3.3
Total	30	100

How were instruments sterilized? Already	13	43.3
Alcohol	2	6.7
Heated	3	10.0
Washed	3	10.0
Machine	8	26.7
Others	1	3.3
Total	30	100

Table 2 above indicates that the highest number of mothers delivered from the hospital 83.3 % (25/30), only one mother reports to have been helped by the traditional birth attendant in her delivery 3.3 % (1/30), and 10.0 % (3/30) delivered from homes 2 from their husband's home while one from the parents' home. 70.0 % (21/30) of the mothers were assisted by the midwives, 10.0% (3/30) were assisted by the doctors, 6.7% (2/30) were assisted by the traditional birth attendants and 13.3% (4/30) were assisted by other people in community while delivering their current babies. Majority of mothers report that their baby's cords were cut using razor blades which were already sterilized or new from packets, however others did not have knowledge on how the instruments used to cut their baby's cord were sterilized.

Knowledge of breastfeeding mothers on Hygiene of their neonates

The knowledge of breastfeeding mothers on hygiene of their neonates was assessed by asking questions on how breastfeeding mothers take care of their neonates from the time of delivery till 28days of the baby's life. Table 3 below shows the findings on questions asked to breastfeeding mothers towards the hygiene of their neonates.

Variable item	Frequency	Percentage
What was put on the cord immediately after delivery? Alcohol	2	6.7
Baby oil	24	80.0
Cow dung	1	3.3
Herbal remedies	1	3.3
Others	2	6.7
Total	30	100
Drinking water be kept in? Any container	8	26.7

Clean covered container	19	63.3
Others	3	10.0
Total	30	100
Young babies sleep in? Clean and dry bed sheets	6	20.0
Clean, dry and ironed bed sheets	22	73.3
Any bed sheet	2	6.7
Total	30	100
How often do baby's bed sheets washed? The bed sheets do not need washing	4	13.3
The bed sheets are long term ones, they don't need washing	3	10.0
I wash the bed sheet whenever I see them dirty	11	36.7
I wash bed sheets every day	9	30.0
Others	3	10.0

Total	30	100
How do you keep toilet? Clean	15	50.0
Covered with a lid	5	16.7
Has water for cleaning	5	16.7
Has brush for cleaning	4	13.3
Not applicable	1	3.3
Total	30	100
How often do baby's utensils washed? After every giving a meal	6	20.0
Twice a day	12	40
Per day	5	16.7
It depends	2	6.7
I don't	5	16.7
Total	30	100

How often do you change diapers? Once a day	8	26.7
When full	5	16.7
I clean and put back	2	6.7
I don't use diapers	10	33.3
When necessary	4	13.3
Total	30	100
How does baby's cord cared of? Clean the cord with salty water	16	53.3
Clean cord with soapy water	7	23.3
Clean cord with plain water	2	6.7
Others	5	16.7
Total	30	100
How mother bathes the baby? With soap and water then dry	12	40.0

Soapy water only	10	33.3
Plain water and dry	6	20.0
With plain water only	2	6.7
Total	30	100
How prepare breast before breastfeeding? Clean water and dry	9	30.0
Just wipe with clean cloth	17	56.7
Just breast feed without clean	1	3.3
Don't breast feed	2	6.7
Others	1	3.3
Total	30	100
How keep child from dust? Keep in clean environment	8	26.7
Rap in clean bed sheets	21	70.0
Just leave anywhere	1	3.3

Total	30	100
Why important to dry baby after bathing? Not applicable	5	16.7
It's not important	1	3.3
To keep baby clean	16	53.3
To prevent diseases and improve hygiene of the baby	8	26.7
Total	30	100

On discharge from the maternity home, mothers are always advised to take care of their baby's cords. However, some mothers do not follow what they were advised to do. The assessment of knowledge of breastfeeding mothers on hygiene of the neonates showed that 80 % (24/30) applied baby oil, 6.7 %(2/30) used alcohol, 3.3%(1/30) applied cow dung, 3.3%(1/30) used herbal remedies in care of their baby's cords. Majority of mothers 73.3% (22/30) rap their babies in clean, dry and ironed bed sheets, 20% rap them in just dry and clean bed sheets while the rest of the population just use any bed sheet. About 53.3 % (16/30) of the mothers knew that the baby's cord is cleaned with saline water, 40.0% reported to bathe their neonates with soapy water and dry, majority 56.7% (12/30) new that the mother's breast should first be wiped before breastfeeding. Concerning the prevention of diseases in babies, 53.3% of mothers reported that it is important to dry the baby after bathing though they did not give a clear reason as to why, while 26.7% of the participants explained why their babies should be dried after bathing as this keeps the baby clean and prevents infections. Majority of mothers 33.3 % (10/30) do not use diapers and those who use diapers always change them whenever they are full.

Practice on hygiene of breast-feeding mothers towards their neonates

The practice of breast-feeding mothers towards the hygiene of their neonates was assessed basing on activities done by mothers when maintaining hygiene of their neonates. Table 4 represents activities done by mothers while maintaining hygiene of their neonates.

Variable items	Frequency	Percentage
What do you use to bathe baby? Only water	2	6.7
Water and soap	20	66.7
Water and oil	2	6.7
Others	6	20.0
Total	30	100

What do you apply on baby's skin? Nothing	5	16.7
Baby oil	16	53.3
Soap	1	3.3
others	8	26.7
Total	30	100
What do you apply on baby's cord? Oil	3	10
Salty water	12	40
Herbs	3	10
Others	12	40
Total	30	100
What do you use to clean baby's cord? Only water	8	26.7
Salty water	9	30

Herbs	12	40
Others	1	3.3
Total	30	100
When do you change diapers when full? Change it when full	21	70
Clean and put back	5	16.7
Don't change till evening	2	6.7
Do not use diapers	2	6.7
Total	30	100
What to do before breastfeed? Nothing	9	30.0
First clean breast	14	46.7
First wash hands	6	20.0
Others	1	3.3
Total	30	100

What do you use when cleaning baby's utensils? Only water	2	6.7
Soap and water	19	63.3
Just wipe	1	3.3
Others	8	26.7
Total	30	100
What use when cleaning baby's linen? Water and soap	27	90.0
Hot water and soap	3	10.0
Total	30	100

Majority of mothers 66.7% (20/30) while practicing hygiene of their neonates, bathe their babies with soap and water, then after 53.3 % (11/30) apply baby oil on the baby's skin in order to keep them clean and moist. 12% of the mothers used normal saline while cleaning their babies' cords and 12% applied normal saline as a maintenance measure for keeping the cord free from infections. About 90% (27/30) reported to at least have washed their baby's linen with water and soap, dry them and iron. Majority of mothers 70% reported that they do not change their babies' diapers until they are full, while others who use diapers 16.7%, they just clean them and put them back.

Qualitative data findings

The qualitative findings from the interviews of 10 (ten) lactating mothers and (3) three focus group discussions revealed a wide range of knowledge and hygiene behavior among the study participants in neonatal care. A few mothers had poor knowledge and unhygienic behavior, while some had good knowledge and frequent hygienic behavior. However, aggregate results reveal significant gaps in awareness, particularly in areas of umbilical cord care, washing of hands before breastfeeding, and general hygiene of neonatal possessions such as clothing, feeding bottles, and bedding.

Some mothers candidly admitted during interviews that they were unsure of correct practices in maintaining their newborn's hygiene. As one mother commented, "I didn't know I had to wash my hands every time before breastfeeding.". I just figured because I shower in the morning, I'm clean enough for the baby during the day." Others reflected this perception in both group and individual interviews, citing the lack of continued reinforcement of hygiene education post-delivery. Another participant indicated that she had received absolutely no neonatal hygiene education, saying, "The nurses were too busy.". They only talked about breastfeeding but not about how to keep the baby clean." During one of the focus group discussions, one of the respondents shared her struggle to keep the surroundings of the baby clean due to a lack of water and soap. She explained, "At home, sometimes we do not have plenty of water even to bathe ourselves properly.".

So, I just use a clean cloth to wipe the baby." Her story provided the backdrop for a broader group discussion about environmental and socio-economic determinants of unhygienic conditions, such as lack of clean water, overcrowded living conditions, and limited access to hygiene products like baby wipes, antiseptic solutions, or disposable nappies.

Cord care was one area where knowledge gaps were extremely evident. Some mothers discussed traditional practices that were opposite to modern medical advice. One participant confessed, "My mother-in-law told me to apply cow ghee and ash to the umbilical cord so that it would fall off earlier.". I was not aware that it would cause an infection." One responded, "I only cleaned the cord when I saw blood or pus, otherwise I thought touching it would be worse." These responses indicated the influence of cultural beliefs and absence of clear advice from health professionals on cord care. Conversely, there was some demonstration of good understanding of hygienic measures by some mothers, which they attributed to previous health education sessions or past experience in childcare. One participant proudly stated, "I always wash my hands with soap before breastfeeding or handling the baby.". I also clean the baby's clothes every day and make sure the bedding is dry and neat." However, even among the knowledgeable mothers, consistent practice remained a challenge due to fatigue, lack of support at home, and sometimes misconceptions. For instance, a mother who initially seemed knowledgeable later admitted, "Sometimes I am too tired to wash my hands after cooking or changing the baby's diaper. I just wipe with a cloth and continue."

In a very perceptive focus group discussion, the mothers felt frustrated at the lack of follow-up and support from the hospital after discharge. As one exclaimed, "After we have given birth, we are discharged so quickly. There is nobody to see if we are doing everything correctly.". Even when we come for immunization, no one talks about hygiene again." This perception was shared, reflecting a gap in postnatal care services, specifically in the delivery of continued health education and practical demonstrations. A few of the participants discussed consulting older family members, which sometimes resulted in contradictory advice. As one explained, "My aunt told me to bathe the baby with herbal water. The midwife told me to bathe the baby with plain warm water only. I was confused about who to believe." This tension between traditional knowledge and biomedical counsel illustrates the need for culturally responsive education that is respectful of local beliefs and still promotes evidence-based practice.

Discussion

This chapter discusses the research findings in relation to the problem statement, literature review of studies conducted elsewhere and in line with the specific study objectives. It also explains the obtained results from the study. Neumann's theory was adopted to describe how mothers respond to their stressors. This theory covers an individual's intrapersonal stressors (physiological, psychological, socio-cultural and spiritual), interpersonal stressors (being away from the family) and extra personal stressors (aggression and psychological pressure) who provide a full concept that affect the client's health.

Knowledge of breastfeeding mothers on hygiene of their neonates

Interview results, focus group discussions, and quantitative data reflect extreme variation in knowledge and hygiene practices among neonatal lactating mothers. Although a minority of mothers practiced exemplary knowledge such as frequent hand washing before breastfeeding, proper cleaning of neonatal garments, and a clean sleeping place a majority practiced minimal knowledge, especially in essential areas such as umbilical cord care, hand washing, and baby bedding and feeding bottle cleanliness.

These findings are consistent with a study in eastern Uganda, which reported that newborn care practices remain poorly performed even where there is availability of health services(Peter Waiswa, 2010). Participants frequently reported lack of awareness or misperception of basic hygiene practices. A mother, for example, did not feel that she needed to wash her hands before every breastfeeding since she bathed in the morning displaying a lack of appreciation for environmental day-to-day contamination risks. The majority of mothers indicated that healthcare providers only focused on breastfeeding education during postnatal care and had no or little neonatal hygiene emphasis. This is supported by a UNICEF report that chronicles the lack of formal postnatal follow-up and health education, leaving the mothers poorly equipped to take care of their newborns(data.unicef.org, 2019; UNICEF, 2017). Environmental and socioeconomic factors were also key drivers of hygiene behavior. One mother in one of the focus groups explained how, due to lack of water, she had washed her baby with a cloth rather than bathing. Other mothers reported similar challenges: overcrowded homes, no availability of antiseptics, baby wipes, or disposable nappies. Such limitations in resources are not new to this study.

Poor knowledge regarding umbilical cord care was a universal theme in all sources of data. Traditional methods such as applying cow ghee, ash, or even dry cow dung to the cord were reported. These practices have a high risk of infection. One mother stated that she only washed the cord when it was bloody or when oozing pus, a central knowledge gap around dry cord care. These findings are consistent with a 2024 study in southwestern Uganda, which found that caregivers commonly applied harmful substances to the cord because healthcare workers failed to offer clear guidance (Happiness P. Sabina, 2025).

Some of the mothers, however, exhibited high levels of awareness, attributing this to past child care experience or exposure to health education by means of clinics or sensitization campaigns in the community. According to one of the respondents, she washed her hands prior to holding her baby and ensured that all bedding was washed and sun-dried. Even well-educated mothers, however, failed to exercise consistency. Lack of support, fatigue, and misinformation were some of the reasons cited for inconsistency. For example, a mother reported that at times she skipped hand washing after cooking or after diaper changes because she was fatigued merely wiping her hands before handling the baby. This shows that knowledge alone is insufficient, mothers require ongoing reinforcement and encouragement to follow hygiene procedures.

Lack of routine postnatal follow-up was a frequent common complaint. Most of the mothers complained that they were dumped after hospital discharge. Though they visited for immunization check-ups, neonatal hygiene was rarely discussed during these visits. It is frustrating, a mother said, that no one visited to inform her that she should practice as instructed. This concurs with WHO's observation that premature discharge without orderly follow-up undermines a mother's capacity to comply with newborn care recommendation(WHO, 2024).

Cultural forces and family pressure also intervened. Conflict advice from professionals and elders confused some of the mothers. For instance, whereas a midwife had advised bath water with kindness, a relative had demanded herbal water. Such advice conflicts caused confusion. Such conflict between old ways and new medicine is so common that culturally appropriate health education that combines local beliefs with safer practices is crucial. Involving elders and community health workers in neonatal hygiene education would be able to bridge this gap.

Additionally, maternal attributes age, level of education, and employment status were identified to affect hygiene knowledge and practice. Older and more educated mothers were likely to possess improved hygiene knowledge, perhaps as a result of experience and higher exposure to health information. Yet, work tended to constrain mothers' time to practice good hygiene on a regular basis. These findings are consistent with those from Kenyatta Hospital, where less-educated and primiparous mothers had worse hygiene knowledge(Amolo L, 2017).

The research also came to find that attendance of ANC was an important indicator of maternal knowledge. Mothers who had ANC from maternity homes or hospitals were instructed in newborn care, while those who did not attend or gave birth with traditional birth attendants relied on the instruction of elders, friends, or community health teams. Thus, 16.7% of mothers in this study indicated the use of unhygienic means of umbilical cord cleaning. Importantly, 3.3% of the mothers used dry cow dung, 3.3% used herbal drugs such as kyogero, and others used ghee, ash, or millet powder. These differ from WHO standards in neonatal hygiene(WHO, 2020) and increase the risks of infection.

To this end, a rural Sierra Leone study showed that mothers' understanding of neonatal hygiene was primarily influenced by health worker advice at antenatal, postnatal, and immunization clinics(Joseph Sam Kanu, 2014). The same pattern was observed in our results, highlighting the importance of healthcare interactions in influencing maternal behavior. Despite challenges, the majority of the mothers in this research acknowledged their babies' vulnerability and had a desire to remain clean. For instance, 73.3% of the mothers wrapped their babies in clean, dry, and ironed bed sheets, and 20% wrapped them in clean but not ironed sheets. The rest wrapped any available piece of material. Poor socioeconomic status was still a major constraint, however.

In addition, whereas 53.3% of mothers indicated drying their babies following a bath, only 26.7% were able to state why. This ignorance was significant considering drying a baby following a bath is crucial to avert bacterial overgrowth in folds of the skin and to keep the baby comfortable and resting. UNICEF (2019) states that drying the baby after a bath keeps the baby calm and avoids skin infections and complications like nappy rash(data.unicef.org, 2019).

Practice of Breastfeeding mothers on neonatal hygiene

During one of the focus group interviews, a respondent described how hard it was to maintain cleanliness around the baby because she had no water and soap. She went on, “At home, at times we do not have much water even to bathe ourselves properly.” So, I simply clean the baby with a clean cloth. “Her evidence evoked a broader discussion surrounding environmental and socio-economic determinants of unhygienic conditions, such as unavailability of clean water, high population living conditions, and limited access to hygiene items like baby wipes, antiseptic liquids, or disposable nappies. Research has uncovered that the mothers from lower socio-economic segments, typically living in rural areas, are prevented from practicing proper hygiene for babies due to limited resources like soap and baby linen (Devendra Raj Singh, 2019). This resource shortage tremendously inhibits their ability to embrace proper neonatal care practices, which might leave babies at higher risks of infections.

Cord care was one area where knowledge gaps were extremely evident. Some mothers discussed traditional practices that contradicted Morden medical advice. One of the respondents confessed, “My mother-in-law told me to apply cow ghee and ash to the umbilical cord so that it would fall off earlier. I did not realize that it would cause infection.” Another answered, “I simple washed the cord only when I saw blood or pus, otherwise, I did not want it to be worse if I touched it”. These responses indicated the dominant influence of the cultural beliefs and insufficient instructions from the health workers on cord care. This is in line with WHO guidance, which advocated cord cleaning using sterile saline and not closing the cord to prevent infection (WHO, 2024).

Alternatively, some evidence of good hygiene practice awareness was found in that some mothers demonstrated that they understood because they had prior health education or prior experience of childcare. One of the women boasted, “I always use soap to wash my hands prior to breastfeeding or handling the baby. I also wash the baby’s clothes every day and ensure that the baby’s beddings are dry and tidy” However, even among the educated mothers, practice became a habit hard to follow due to fatigue, home lack of support, and occasional misconceptions. For example, one of the mothers who seemed to be pretty well-educated on initial impression admitted, "Sometimes I am too exhausted to wash my hands after preparing food or changing the baby's diaper. I simply wipe with a cloth and carryon"

One particularly insightful focus group session saw the mothers vent about the absence of follow- up and support from the hospital after discharge. One mother exclaimed, "After we have given birth, we are dispatched so soon. There is no one to watch whether we do things correctly. Even if we come back for immunization, nobody ever talks about hygiene again." This phrase is an indicator of an absence of coverage of postnatal care services, specifically om the form pf continuous health education and demonstration. A few respondents also stated seeking counsel from elder relatives, sometimes leading to contradictory advice. Once mother said, "My aunt instructed me to wash the baby with herbal water. The midwife instructed me to wash the baby with plain warm water alone. I was in conflict about whom to trust." This conflict between local knowledge and biomedical advice indicates the necessity of culturally responsive education that honors local belief while encouraging evidence-based practice in neonatal cleanliness.

The research showed that although the majority of the mothers in the community understood the importance of baby hygiene, others were still unable to employ the correct steps. The study uncovered that a simple 66.7% of the mothers washed the babies with soap, water and baby oil, whereas 33.3% washed the babies with water alone(Devendra Raj Singh, 2019). Further, the survey also found improper hygienic practice for diaper, skin, and cord care, thus exposing the neonates to infection. Only 12% employed saline water as a cleansing solution for the umbilical cords of their babies, and only 12% employed normal saline as a temporary measure in keeping the health of the umbilical region free from infection as per WHO recommendations (WHO, 2020, 2024). Furthermore, 70% of the mothers indicated not disposing of their infants' diapers until they were full, and 16.7% of the diaper users cleaned the diapers and reused them. General recommendations for diaper usage indicate that neonates need diaper changes every 2 to 3 hours because they tend to urinate frequently (UNICEF, 2018). This highlights the necessity for or education and resources to enable mothers to be able to apply the appropriate hygiene practices to their neonates so as to avert infection and proper growth.

Conclusion

The study involved 30 mothers for quantitative survey, 10 mothers for in-depth interviews plus 5 group focused discussions from post-natal and immunization clinics from Mukono General Hospital in the month of November, 2020. Most of the mothers were first time mothers with babies below 28days. The modal age group was between 20 to 24 years, a reflection of national peak fertility age in both urban and rural areas of Uganda. Uganda's most recent demographic survey indicated fertility rate in Kampala metropolitan to be 2 children per woman.

Maternal knowledge and practice on neonatal hygiene was influenced by individual characteristics of the mother and perinatal preparation of the health workers. Knowledge and practice gaps on hygiene of neonates were however identified in the study. Some mothers were not aware of proper hygiene practices towards heir neonates and those who knew were unable to practice what they know.

Health workers give enough information on pamper use, cord and skin care during postnatal and immunization clinics however some mothers said that the midwives did not give them time. Most mothers had knowledge on proper care of cord and skin plus pamper however their practice was affected by some barriers like low socioeconomic status and overwhelming responsibilities.

Recommendations

Health workers need to bridge the gap between the community and health workers to encourage mothers seek healthcare freely without fear.

The ministry of health needs to evaluate the effectiveness of hygiene support provided by the health workers at health facilities to determine whether proper hygiene education needs strengthening.

There is a need to sensitize and guide the community on proper hygiene practices towards maternal and child health.

The ministry of health needs to involve traditional birth attendants and village health teams in enforcing the guidelines of World Health Organization on child and maternal care.

Work was identified as one of the barriers to the practice of hygiene of breastfeeding mothers towards their neonates. Employers need to be sensitized and guided more on the support of breastfeeding mothers.

Practices of some mothers on neonatal hygiene were affected by low socioeconomic status of the mothers. Male individuals need to be sensitized and guided on the support of their wives during and after their pregnancy.

There is a need to empower single mothers through microfinance businesses to enable them earn a living and support their families.

There is also a need for sensitizing the adolescent girls and the community as a whole on the relevance of preparedness before pregnancy.

The ministry of health needs to increase on the sensitization of the community about family planning use to prevent unwanted pregnancies.

Limitation

The outbreak of Covid-19 disease in the country which was spreading at a high rate with high mortality and morbidity rate, made the sample size small because of health ministry standard operating procedures which discouraged mass gathering.

Acknowledgement

We are so grateful to all those who have helped us and also continued to support us in the journey of writing this proposal. We cannot mention each person but we are greatly indebted to our supervisor, Mercy Muwema Mwanja for her invaluable input and guidance in writing this proposal for the basis of research writing, together with friends for their time in proposal development.

To Madam Namara Alex Lwasa (senior nursing officer of Mukono general hospital), we appreciate your support and commitment through the process of getting the study site. Thank you very much.

Definition of Terms

A **neonate** is a newborn not exceeding 28 days of life (WHO, 2010)

Breast feeding is the provision of nourishment to children through breast milk by direct suckling or of expressed human milk through any other means (WHO, 2003)

Environmental factors are external features of a person's environment (J Fooken. 2016).

Hygiene is the practice or principles of keeping the body and environment clean in order to maintain health and prevent diseases (Arisa, 2014)

Knowledge is the awareness of someone or something such as facts, information, descriptions which is acquired through experience, education, discovering or learning (oxford dictionary).

Mortality is the measure of the number of deaths in a particular population, scaled to the size of that population, per unit of time (WHO, 2020).

Mother is the woman who gives birth or who has the responsibility of physical and emotional care for specific children (Cambridge dictionary)

Neonatal mortality rate is the death of children during the first 28days of life (UNICEF, 2019).

Physiological factors are factors related to physical body that affect functioning (J Fooken. 2016).

Practice is the use of an idea (Oxford dictionary, eighth edition)

Socioeconomic factors these are factors that relate to and influence one another (J Fooken. 2016)

Abbreviations

AIDS-Acquired Immune Deficiency Syndrome

ANC-Antenatal Care

BMC-Biomed Central

HIV-Human Immune Deficiency Virus

IDP-Internally Displaced Persons

MOH- Ministry of Health

NMR-Neonatal Mortality Rate

PPH-Post Partum Hemorrhage

SPSS-Statistical Package of Social Sciences

TBA-Traditional Birth Attendants

UNICEF-United Nations Children's Fund

WHO- World Health Organization

References

Amanuel Nuramo Sakelo, N. A., Lemessa Oljira, and Zebene Mekonnen Assefa. (2020). Newborn Care Practice and Associated Factors among Mothers of One-Month-Old Infants in Southwest Ethiopia. https://doi.org/https://doi.org/10.1155/2020/3897427

Amolo L, I. G., Njai D. (2017). Knowledge of postnatal mothers on essential newborn care practices at the Kenyatta National Hospital: a cross sectional study. https://doi.org/10.11604/pamj.2017.28.97.13785

Annettee Nakimuli, S. N. M., Rose C Nabirye, Othman Kakaire, Sarah Nakubulwa, Michael O Osinde, Nelson Kakande4 and Dan K Kaye. (2015). Still births, neonatal deaths and neonatal near miss cases attributable to severe obstetric complications: a prospective cohort study in two referral hospitals in Uganda. 8. https://doi.org/10.1186/s12887-015-0362-3

data.unicef.org. (2019). *Levels & Trends in Estimates developed by the United Nations Inter-agency Group for Child Mortality Estimation. Child Mortality.*

Devendra Raj Singh, C. M. H., Pushpalata Bohara, Dhirendra Nath, Sunita Singh, Sylvia Szabo, Kshitij Karki. (2019). Factors associated with newborn care knowledge and practices in the upper Himalayas. https://doi.org/10.1371/journal.pone.0222582

Happiness P. Sabina, N. S. M., Bumani S. Manganye. (2025). Home-based care for umbilical cords of neonates by family caregivers in Mpumalanga province, South Africa.

Jacob Sandberg, K. O. P., Gustav Asp, Jerome Kabakyenga, Anette Agardh. (2014). Inadequate Knowledge of Neonatal Danger Signs among Recently Delivered Women in Southwestern Rural Uganda: A Community Survey. https://doi.org/10.1371/journal.pone.0097253

Joseph Sam Kanu, Y. T., Yawen Liu. (2014). Assessment on the Knowledge and Reported Practices of Women on Maternal and Child Health in Rural Sierra Leone: A Cross-Sectional Survey. https://doi.org/10.1371/journal one.0105936

Peter Waiswa, S. P., Goran Tomson, George W Pariyo. (2010). Poor newborn care practices - a population based survey in eastern Uganda. 8. https://doi.org/http://www.biomedcentral.com/1471-2393/10/9

Saadia Gul, R. K., M.Tahir Yousafzai, Faiza Shoukat. (2014). Newborn care knowledge and practices among mothers attending pediatric outpatient clinic of a hospital in Karachi, Pakistan. *8*, 9.

UDHS, U. B. O. S. (2015). National Population and Housing Census 2014.

UDHS, U. B. O. S. (2023). *Uganda Demographic Health Survey*.

UNICEF. (2017). https://www.unicef.org/uganda/key-practice-newborn-care

UNICEF. (2018). Newborn Care Practices. https://www.unicef.org/uganda/key-practice-newborn-care

WHO, W. H. O. (2020, 20th, October,2024). Newborns: improving survival and well-being. https://www.who.int/en/news-room/fact-sheets/detail/newborns-reducing-mortality

WHO, W. H. O. (2024). *Neonatal Mortality* https://www.who.int/news-room/fact-sheets/detail/newborn-mortality

More Books!

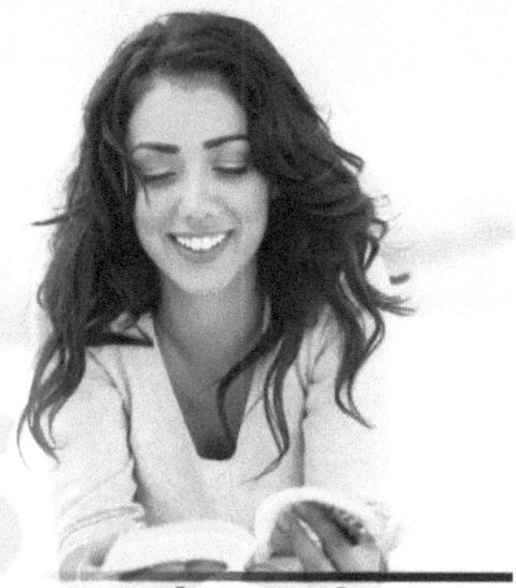

I want morebooks!

Buy your books fast and straightforward online - at one of world's fastest growing online book stores! Environmentally sound due to Print-on-Demand technologies.

Buy your books online at
www.morebooks.shop

Kaufen Sie Ihre Bücher schnell und unkompliziert online – auf einer der am schnellsten wachsenden Buchhandelsplattformen weltweit! Dank Print-On-Demand umwelt- und ressourcenschonend produzi ert.

Bücher schneller online kaufen
www.morebooks.shop

info@omniscriptum.com
www.omniscriptum.com

OMNIScriptum

FSC
www.fsc.org
MIX
Papier | Fördert
gute Waldnutzung
FSC® C083411

Kolibri 360 GmbH
Ferdinand-Jühlke-Straße 7
99095 Erfurt, Deutschland
produktsicherheit@kolibri360.de

Druck:
CPI Druckdienstleistungen GmbH
im Auftrag der
Kolibri 360 GmbH
Ferdinand-Jühlke-Str. 7
99095 Erfurt